Hip Pain

Treating Hip Pain
Preventing Hip Pain
All Natural Remedies For Hip Pain
Medical Cures For Hip Pain
Along With Exercises And Rehab For
Hip Pain Relief

By Ace McCloud
Copyright © 2014

Disclaimer

The information provided in this book is designed to provide helpful information on the subjects discussed. This book is not meant to be used, nor should it be used, to diagnose or treat any medical condition. For diagnosis or treatment of any medical problem, consult your own physician. The publisher and author are not responsible for any specific health or allergy needs that may require medical supervision and are not liable for any damages or negative consequences from any treatment, action, application or preparation, to any person reading or following the information in this book. Any references included are provided for informational purposes only. Readers should be aware that any websites or links listed in this book may change.

Table of Contents

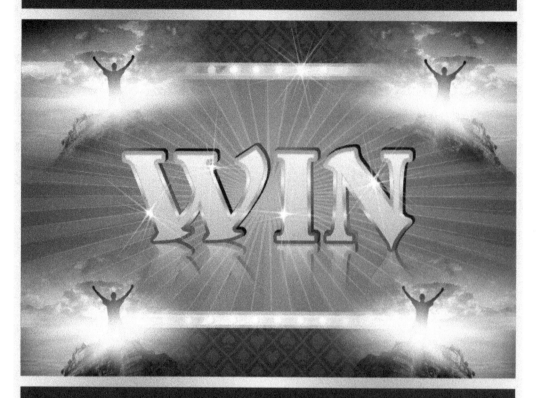

Be sure to check out my website for all my Books and Audio books.

www.AcesEbooks.com

Introduction

I want to thank you and congratulate you for buying the book, "Hip Pain Cure: How To Treat Hip Pain, How To Prevent Hip Pain, All Natural Remedies For Hip Pain, Medical Cures For Hip Pain, Along With Exercises and Rehab For Hip Pain Relief."

This book contains proven steps and strategies on how to treat hip pain from injuries or aging and how to stop it from occurring altogether. You will learn about the different causes of hip pain, as well as how to stretch and exercise to keep your hips healthy throughout your entire life. For those already suffering from hip pain, you will read about the different medical and all-natural ways to treat hip pain, including some of the best products you can use. This book will also introduce you to a variety of exercises that you can use to rehabilitate yourself if you've incurred a hip injury and teach you the proper ways to stretch your hips for flexibility and pain relief. Finally, you will learn about a variety of ways to stay motivated throughout the process of strengthening your hips!

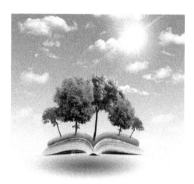

Chapter 1: Understanding Your Hips, Hip Pain, and Hip Injuries

Your hips are one of the biggest joints in your body. Some call it a ball-and-socket joint. A band of tissue called your ligaments keeps the ball connected to the socket, which helps keep your hips stable. The joint is covered by a cartilage known as articular cartilage. The hip joint is also covered by a thin tissue, which helps reduce friction and keeps your cartilage lubricated. Your hips are a very important part of your body—they help you engage in repeated motions, like running, and they help your body move in general.

Although your hips are durable, they are not immune from damage, deterioration, or injury. Like any part of your skeleton, the cartilage on your hips can be worn down, you can overuse the muscle, or you can fracture it in an impact injury. Wear and tear or injuries to your hips can eventually cause hip pain. Hip pain affects many people, young and old, all over the world. The elderly population has the highest risk of incurring bad hip injuries and feeling hip pain because of the wear and tear they have placed on their hips throughout their entire life. Athletes and those who regularly play contact sports also have a high risk of incurring a hip injury or feeling hip pain due to injuries or excessive overuse.

The good news is that there are ways to protect and strengthen your hips against injuries and the effects of aging. Most of the strategies explained in this book revolve around general health and many of the exercises and stretches also benefit other areas of the body besides your hips, so by taking care of your hips you can also take care of your body at the same time.

The Signs and Symptoms of Hip Pain

When you are experiencing pain in your hips, there is likely something wrong with them. However, if you are experiencing hip pain, it is possible to also feel pain in your thigh, groin, buttocks, and on each side of your hip, making your entire body feel very uncomfortable. Hip pain may even be caused by another nearby body part. If your hips begin to ache while you are actively doing something, there is a good chance that they may be affected by arthritis or an injury.

What Conditions Can Cause Hip Pain?

There are several fairly common causes of hip pain, ranging from impact injuries to deterioration. This section will give you a brief overview of some of the main sources of hip pain. You can use this section to determine if you think you have or are prone to developing hip pain.

Arthritis is one of the major sources of hip pain. Senior citizens are especially prone to developing arthritis of the hips. Arthritis causes your hip joints to become inflamed, which then damages the cartilage that keeps your hip bones padded. If left untreated, the pain can slowly worsen. Arthritis can cause your hips to become tight and can limit your range of motion. **Post Traumatic Arthritis** can also occur following a serious fracture.

Bone Cancer may be one cause of hip pain. When cancerous tumors develop or spread to your hip bone, you will be able to feel it. However, bone cancer can cause pain in all of your bones so it is important to consult with a doctor if you believe that you have bone cancer.

Bursitis is another condition that can cause hip pain. This condition occurs if you repeat an activity so much that it overworks your hip bone. When this happens, the fluid-filled sacs that keep your tendons and muscles safe become inflamed.

Fractures are the second most common cause of hip pain. Once again, senior citizens are especially susceptible to incurring a hip bone fractured due to aging bones. The weaker your bones are, the more likely they will break during an impact or fall.

Stress Fractures, which are fractures that develop over time, can cause hip pain in athletes who consistently use their hip bones. Stress fractures are caused by weight that is put on your lower body each day and can be affected by your diet as well. Women who have irregular periods are also susceptible to hip stress fractures. If you are an athlete who feels pain in the hip after starting a work out, you may have a stress fracture.

Contusions occur when your hip incurs a direct blow from a contact sport or other similar circumstance. Hockey and football are two of the most common sports in which hip contusions happen. In mild hip contusions, sometimes your hip will only be bruised. A severe hip contusion can lead to a fracture. Both will cause pain.

Dislocations are another type of injury that may cause hip pain. If your hips are dislocated, it means that one or more of your bones is not aligned with your body the way it should be. A fall or an impact injury can also cause a dislocation. Dislocations often cause immediate pain, swelling, and limited movement. A dislocated hip bone is considered an emergency.

Osteonecrosis is a condition in which blood does not flow to your hip bones, and this is another common cause of hip pain. Without the proper flow of blood, the tissue on your hip bone can die, possibly causing pain. This condition can stem from a fracture or from using too many high-dosage steroids.

General strain can cause hip pain without inflaming the sacs around your tendons and muscles. For example, if you overwork your hips from running too much, they may start to ache.

Finally, **childhood disease** can also be a factor in hip pain. Sometimes, your hip will not grow as it should when you are a child or a baby. Most often, hip problems can be solved during your adolescence, but it may lead to hip pain later in life.

Chapter 2: How To Prevent Hip Pain Before It Happens

While injuries can often be preventable (but not always), aging and deterioration of your hips is often hard to avoid. However, the good news is that as long as you take good care of your hips, as well as every other part of your body, those body parts will perform better for much longer. This chapter will teach you about some different types of stretches and strength training exercises that you can integrate into your daily routine to help maintain your hips over time.

Stretching

To prevent hip pain and hip injuries, stretching is a must. Stretching helps your hips become more flexible and more resistant to injuries in the event of a car accident, sports injury, fall, or other impact. Moreover, getting into the habit of stretching as soon as you can may help prevent the onset of hip pain as you get older.

One good way to stretch your hips is to do the **bridge stretch**. The bridge stretch is a good thing to start your day off with so that you can have fluid movement throughout the day. To start this exercise, lie on the ground face-up, bringing your knees up while keeping your feet on the floor. Also, make sure that your feet are aligned with your hips. Press down on the floor with your feet and bring your buttocks up as you tighten your stomach muscles. Try to bring your body into a position where it creates a straight line from your chest to your knees. Hold the position for 5 seconds and slowly bring yourself back down. You can do this stretch in 10 repetitions. This stretch is a little different from the yoga bridge pose so to see it in action, please check out this YouTube video by Josh Schlottman, Trainer Josh Fixes Low Back Pain: Hip Bridge Progressions.

Another good type of stretch is called the **hip rotation**. A hip rotation can strengthen the range of motion on either side of your hips. To do this, bend one of your legs with your accompanying foot flat on the floor, while keeping your other leg in place with your toes pointing upwards. Slowly begin to rotate your bent knee by bringing it away from your body, as comfortably as you can. Hold the stretch for 5 seconds and then come back. Do this 10 times for each side. For a visual demonstration, check out this YouTube video, How To Increase Golf Swing Speed – Hip Rotation Stretch Tip by Perform Better Golf.

A third good type of stretch is called the **hip flexion**. The hip flexion strengthens your range of motion, like the hip rotation stretch, but it also helps reduce any stiffness. To do this, lie on the ground and fully stretch your legs out. Bend one of your legs and pull your knee as close to your body as you comfortably can. Hold the stretch for five seconds and then return to your original position. You can do this 10 times for each leg.

The stretch known as the **gluteal squeeze** works both your hips and your inner thighs. This stretch can help you build up strength to protect yourself against any injuries. For this stretch, you will need a foam roller or a tightly rolled towel. Lie on your back and bend your knees with your feet on the floor. Place the foam roller or the towel between your two knees and squeeze them together, holding it for five seconds. Let go and repeat. You can do this 10 times.

Hip Strengthening Exercises

The Single Leg Hip Lift is a great exercise to start out with. To do this, lie on the floor and bend your legs at your knees. Lift one foot up, along with your hips, push with your heels and let your gluteal muscles contract. Make sure that you keep your toes pointed up. Hold the stretch for 5 seconds and return to your original position. You can do 2 sets of 10 repetitions. For a visual of this exercise, please check out this YouTube video by diethealth, Single Leg Hip Lifts.

A second hip strength exercise is the **Split Squat.** This exercise is great for stretching your hip flexor and improving hip mobility. Start out by standing with your feet spread wide apart. Shifting all your weight to one side, bring your hips down while keeping your knee bent over your toes. Make sure all your weight is on your bent leg. Allow yourself to stretch for two seconds and then come back, alternating each side. To see this exercise in action, please check out James Wilson's YouTube video Split Squat.

A third great strength exercise to improve motion in your hips is the **Lateral Lunge.** To start, stand with your feet not too wide apart, while keeping your leg straight and then take a step to the side. Be sure to keep your hips back and place your weight on your heels. Also be sure to keep your chest upright. You can do this for 10 repetitions. For a visual of this exercise, please check out this YouTube video.

A fourth great strength increasing exercise for your hips is the **Butterfly Stretch**. This exercise is great for loosening tight hip flexors as well as strengthening your inner thighs and lower back. To do this, sit upright and bring the soles of your feet together. Let your knees bend so that they look like the wings of a butterfly. Next, pull in your stomach muscles and lean in from your hips. Hold your feet with your hands and gently pull yourself forward. Allow yourself to stretch for a few seconds and then let go. To see this exercise in action, please check out this YouTube video by fatlosspro, The Lateral Lunge.

Here are some more excellent strength training exercises to try:

Front to Back Leg Swings

While gripping a stable surface, keep one leg straight and begin swinging the other back and forth. Instead of generating power from your thighs, make sure you generate it from your hip socket so you can work your hips. Also make sure that you keep your back stationary and tight. You should swing each leg back and forth 15 times. To see this exercise in action, check out this YouTube video, Hip Mobility – Front to Back Leg Swings by Mark Young.

Side to Side Leg Swings

This exercise is performed like the front to back leg swings, except you will be swinging your legs from side to side. To prevent yourself from turning your chest, make sure that you lead with your hips and keep them firm. You should also do each leg 15 times.

Fire Hydrants

Get on all fours and keep your hands underneath your shoulders. Keeping your spine neutral, lift each leg up, hold it, and then let it down. Do this 15 times per leg. This exercise works your hip girdle. To see this exercise in action, check out this YouTube video by mahalodotcom, How to Do the Fire Hydrant – Myrtl Exercise for the Hip Girdle.

Reverse Lunge with Twist

Take one step back as far as you can and get down on one knee. Rotate your upper body toward your other knee. This exercise helps you stretch your hip flexors. You should do this ten times for each leg. To see this exercise in action, check out this YouTube video.

Squat Stands

Start this exercise by standing with your feet a little more than shoulder-width apart. Keep your legs straight, touch your toes, and lower yourself into a squatting position. Keep your elbows inside of your knees with your knees positioned over your feet. Then, curve your back, bring your hands over your head, and bring yourself back up. Be sure to curve your back and not to round it, otherwise your hips will not benefit from this exercise. You should do 10 repetitions of this move. To see this exercise in action in a simplified form, check out this YouTube video, How to Do Squat-to-Stands With Overhead Reach by Livestrong.com.

Hip Thrusts

Sit down and let your back rest against a stable surface. With your feet on the floor, keep your knees bent up. Firmly press your feet into the ground, squeeze your glutes, and thrust your hips forward until your chest sticks out. To see this exercise in action, check out this How To: Hip Thrust YouTube video by ScottHermanFitness.

Therapeutic Exercises to Loosen Tight Hips

There are some techniques that you can do every day to keep your hips from becoming too tight. You can do them after exercising, when you get up each day, before going to bed, or you can do them whenever your hips feel tight. All you need is a simple massage tool, like a foam roller or even a tennis ball. If you decide to invest in a foam roller to help loosen up the soft tissue in your body, I highly recommend the Black High Density Foam Roller.

One way to loosen your hips is to massage yourself from the top of your hips to your thigh area. Using a foam roller, roll it down your hips and thighs until you come to your knee. If you roll over any painful areas, stop and hold it there for a few seconds. You can try rolling your foam roller down different angles to see what feels best. For maximum results, try to do this 15 times on each side. To see this exercise in action, check out this YouTube video by BodySpex, Thigh, IT Band myofascial release.

To massage your hip adductors, straddle a foam roller and roll it over your inner thighs, 15 times on each leg. To see this exercise in action, check out this YouTube video, The Squash Secret 7 short adductor/groin foam rolling technique, by TheInspirationhunter. You can also use the foam roller on your hamstring if you want to apply more pressure.

Protective Braces/Wraps

Wearing protective hip braces or wraps can help you stop the onset of hip pain whether you're working out or just engaging in daily activities. These products can help stabilize your hips, which keeps them aligned and pain-free during movement. Protective braces and wraps don't usually restrict your movement and are comfortable to wear underneath your clothes. They are a great investment for keeping your hips strong and stable.

Purchasing a protective hip brace or wrap is relatively inexpensive and can save you a lot of aggravation in the future. Here are some of the best-made products that you can get for your money and health.

The first wrap that is effective yet inexpensive is the OPTP SI-Loc Wrap. This wrap comes in two different sizes—small/medium and large/extra-large. It fits comfortably under your clothes and is made from fabric that doesn't suffocate your skin. It adheres to your body so that it doesn't fall out of place and works great. Just be sure to measure yourself in advance, since this product cannot be returned.

Another option that works just as well is the New Serola SI Support Belt. This belt has a few more size options, ranging from a small hip of up to 34 inches to triple extra-large, so there is a size for everybody. It is specially designed to compress your hip joints for extra stability so that not only do your hips stay strong, but so does your legs and back. This is a really good wrap for those who want to work out after incurring an injury.

Speaking of injuries, if you play impact sports or suffer from ongoing deterioration pain, the last wrap I would highly suggest is the Soft Gel Hip Ice Wrap. I will talk about the benefits of using ice therapy to treat hip pain in a later chapter, but this wrap is really good to keep around the house to quickly and effectively treat hip pain. It wraps right around your body and has a comfortable fit. It stays cold for long time and compresses tightly for deep tissue healing.

Finding a good protective hip brace or wrap is important for protecting your hips in almost any situation. It is a good investment and something that you can keep around your house for any time you may feel hip pain or want to work out while protecting your hips.

Chapter 3: Medical Solutions For Hip Pain

Sometimes, when your pain is severe, it is a good idea to see a doctor about what you can do to treat your hip problems. Your doctor can give you an in-depth examination to help determine exactly what you may need to do in order to help restore your hips. In some mild cases, your doctor may just recommend icing your injury and staying off of it for a while. However, if your hip injury or pain is so severe that it cannot be treated naturally, he or she may recommend that you undergo a medical procedure. This chapter will introduce you to a couple of the most popular and effective medical procedures for eliminating hip pain so you can go into your doctor's appointment knowledgeable and ready to discuss your options.

Laser Surgery

One option for treating hip pain or a hip injury is K-Laser therapy. This type of therapy utilizes an infrared laser to safely, painlessly, and effectively reduce inflammation and pain. It also encourages faster healing of your muscles, ligaments, and tissues. What makes laser therapy unique is that it can target any injured cells in your hip to help them heal faster. If you experience a sprain, strain, impact injury, or if you are developing arthritis, laser surgery can be an easier and more cost-effective alternative to major surgery. Laser surgery also has no side effects and takes up less time than major surgery, so you can have more time to relax and heal. The cost of laser surgery varies depending on your location and your insurance but most specialists charge an average of $40 to $60 per session.

Acupuncture

For those who suffer from arthritis or chronic joint pain in the hips, acupuncture is a good alternative to surgery. Acupuncture has been a medical healing technique in the Chinese culture for thousands of years. During an acupuncture procedure, a practitioner will put small needles in your hips and adjust them as needed to help relieve pain. Acupuncture is safe and some insurance companies even cover it under their medical plans. Even if you're afraid of needles or pain, you don't have to worry, because acupuncture can be very painless when done correctly. The key is to find a reputable practitioner in your area.

Over-The-Counter Solutions

Sometimes, if you are just suffering from a flare up of arthritis or a minor sprain or strain, an over-the-counter pain reliever will do wonders. Common pain relievers such as Tylenol, or Motrin work well. If you're not a fan of taking pills, I highly recommend trying a pain relief ointment called Penetrex. This ointment can be used for almost any type of pain, including arthritis and hip pain. It works great, has a money-back guarantee, and smells pretty good too. It actually helps the body heal injuries, which is why it is so popular.

If you specifically suffer from a form of arthritis but you don't want to shell out the money for multiple laser therapy sessions, another option is to invest in the Tens Electronic Pulse Massager. This small, portable, and safe device utilizes electrical stimulation to help heal and relieve pain. It's a great tool for reliving stiffness or muscle aches.

Rheumatoid Arthritis Treatment

For those who suffer from really severe arthritis in your hip, you may consider looking into rheumatoid arthritis treatment. This type of treatment requires a doctor's evaluation and is best for controlling pain and inflammation. One option in this type of treatment is to take a high-dose non-steroidal anti-inflammatory drug, which you will need a prescription to get. If your arthritis is so bad that those medical drugs cannot help, your doctor may prescribe you a biologic, which is a genetically engineered protein that works with your immune system to reduce pain. However, you should note that one major side effect of biologics is the possibility of an infection. Another option under this treatment is to take steroids. You can take steroids to combat arthritis pain flare ups or to treat extra severe rheumatoid arthritis. Steroids come in the form of an injection or pill, and be sure to talk to your doctor about possible side effects.

Total Hip Replacement

You may consider turning to total hip replacement surgery if your hips are so damaged that you are almost constantly in pain and your medications and exercises are not working. Most people who consider undergoing total hip replacement experience hip pain that interferes with daily living, sleeping comfortably, or limits your ability to be mobile. A total hip replacement surgery is an alternative option that can get you back to normal if everything goes well. Just how safe is a total hip replacement surgery? It's pretty safe, but when things go wrong, the consequences are pretty terrible. Over 285,000 people undergo total hip replacement surgeries each year. Like its name, total hip replacement is the process of removing your original hip and replacing it with an artificial joint. Most often, the artificial parts are made of metal.

The best way to get customized information on how a total hip replacement surgery will affect your life is to speak with your general doctor. Your doctor can most likely refer you to a specialist. Then, you should consult with both your regular doctor, your surgeon, and your family to be sure that it is the right decision for you. Although there have been some cases of successful total hip replacement procedures in young people, most adults who undergo this procedure are between the ages of 50 and 80. The majority of total hip replacement surgeries are based off of individual evaluations.

During an evaluation, you should be prepared to share your medical history with your physician. Also, you should expect to undergo x-rays, a physical, and possibly some other tests, such as an MRI. If you, your doctor, and your family agree that total hip replacement surgery is for you, you may want to consider having handrails, a heightened toilet seat, and safety bars installed in your home to make the recovery process safer and easier.

From personal experience, my father underwent hip replacement surgery a little over a year ago. Everything was fine at the beginning and he recovered nicely. However he developed some problems around six months after the surgery. He was having a large amount of pain where the hip implant was placed. After returning to the doctors they originally misdiagnosed him as having a hematoma on his hip and prescribed physical therapy. Another six months went by with him steadily getting worse. After returning to the doctors it was discovered that the hip was infected with a metal eating bacteria.

So now he has to do another surgery to take out the infected hip implant, clean out the bacteria, while they place a temporary cement implant in his hip treated with medicine to kill any lingering bacteria. Then the doctors will have to check after several months to see if the bacteria has been eliminated. If it hasn't been eliminated then he will have to undergo 1 to 3 more surgeries until the bacteria is totally eliminated and then a final surgery to insert a new hip implant.

My father always complains that he wished he had tried harder to rehab his hips naturally before resorting to surgery. He is now looking at a grueling one-year recovery time with multiple surgeries. While many surgeries are successful, I just wanted to let you know some of the devastating side effects that can happen if it doesn't go well.

Update: After another 6 months and two more surgeries my father has survived but the whole ordeal took a terrible toll on him and his mobility is much worse than if he had done nothing at all. These new antibiotic resistant super bugs in the hospitals can be very dangerous!

Chapter 4: The Best All-Natural Remedies For Hip Pain

Sometimes, all it takes to treat hip pain are some natural, home remedies. Whether it's treating your pain with cold or heat or adding important nutrients to your diet, you can learn how to stay pain-free and out of the doctor's office at the same time. This chapter will take a look at some of the best all-natural and time-tested home remedies for hip pain.

Ice/Heat Therapy

Ice packs or heating pads are one of the best and most common ways to naturally treat hip pain at home. Ice packs are good for reducing any swelling or inflammation of your joints. Heating pads are best for allowing your muscles to relax and encouraging better blood flow. You can easily make an ice compress at home by wrapping ice cubes in a cloth or you can buy an instant icepack, which you can store and use when needed. A really great instant icepack that you can buy is the Dynarex Instant Cold Pack. This product comes with 24 packs, so you can stock up your medicine cabinet for whenever you are in pain. For instant heat therapy, I highly recommend a product called the Thermalon Microwave Activiated Moist Heat Therapy Wrap. This heating pad comes with ties so you can tie it around any part of your body, including your hips. You can generate heat from it by putting it in the microwave and wrapping it around your area of pain. The heat lasts for about 10 to 15 minutes and then you can reheat it if you need more time. The best part about ice or heat therapy is that you can often do it yourself, at home, and on your own schedule.

Omega-3 Fatty Acids

By making sure you get enough omega-3 fatty acids in your diet, you can help relieve hip pain. Omega-3 fatty acids contain anti-inflammatory properties, which can help offset any pain you may be experiencing. Omega-3 fatty acids can also provide nutrients to your heart, brain, and skin, making it an all-around nutrient. Since your body is unable to produce omega-3 fatty acids on its own, you have to get it by either eating fish (salmon, mackerel, and anchovies are the best sources) or by taking a natural supplement. One of the best, most highly recommended omega-3 fatty acids supplement is Kirkland Signature Fish Oil.

Vitamin D and Calcium

Vitamin D and Calcium are crucial in building strong bones, especially hip bones. The proper amount of calcium can help lower your risk of fracturing a bone and vitamin D helps your bones become and stay strong. By ensuring that you get the right amount of these vitamins and minerals in your diet, you can help yourself become more protected in the event of a fall or an injury. You can provide your body with vitamin D by eating egg yolks, liver, fish, or by drinking fortified milk.

You can get calcium by eating cheese, yogurt, salmon, broccoli, or baked beans. Some great supplements to take for vitamin D and calcium are NOW Foods Vitamin D and Nature Made Calcium Magnesium Zinc.

Turmeric

Turmeric is an Asian herb that can help reduce inflammation in your body. A research team at the University of Arizona even did a study on the effects of turmeric and joint inflammation in rats. They found that the rats who were injected with a bacteria and turmeric at the same time suffered from less swelling than the rats that did not receive the turmeric. Many people use turmeric to cook curry, which is an Indian dish. If you don't want to cook with it, you can also take it through a supplement. One of the best turmeric supplements is Swanson Premium Brand Turmeric.

Cherries

Did you know that cherries have anti-inflammatory properties? Studies have shown that if you suffer from arthritis in your hips or if you've pulled a hip muscle, eating cherries can actually help lessen the pain. Specifically, sour and tart cherries are the best for relieving pain. They also serve as an antioxidant, which also helps with pain relief. Best of all, cherries are healthy for your entire body and are delicious at the same time. If you're experiencing hip pain, try to eat some cherries to see if they can help you.

R.I.C.E

If your hip pain stems from a recent injury, one of the most time-tested traditions is to follow the R.I.C.E acronym—Rest, Ice, Compression, and Elevation. You should rest for at least two days following a hip injury to allow it to heal quicker. By icing the injury, you can help reduce the onset of swelling and inflammation. By compressing the injury, usually with an ace bandage, you can help stabilize the injury. Finally, you should elevate your injured hip to relieve any additional pain. It can be challenging to elevate your hips but you can do it by resting with your feet up.

Chapter 5: Stretches and Strength Exercises

Having a plan in place to strengthen and exercise your hips can help you protect them against injuries and other unwanted conditions. It can also help you keep other parts of your body healthy, such as your buttocks, thighs, and back. This chapter will show you an example of a hip conditioning plan that you can use to strengthen your hips if you've been recently injured or in pain. For the best results, try to stick with this program for 4 to 6 weeks. Even if you do not currently have any hip problems, you can still engage in these exercises to keep your hips healthy and strong. By engaging in these exercises for at least 2 days a week, you can maintain strong and flexible hips that can last you a lifetime.

Walking

Walking makes a great warm-up exercise. It's a low-impact activity and easy to do. You can walk for 5 or 10 minutes to get started. You can walk inside on a treadmill or a track or you can take a nice walk in your neighborhood or local park. If you're a person who enjoys walking almost every day, I highly recommend getting some special gel shoe inserts. A great brand to try is Run Pro Insoles. I use these because they help take away the pain in my hips that I felt when I would go on long walks. They also provided great comfort to my knees and ankles.

Swimming

Swimming is a great exercise for strengthening and rehabbing your hips and people of all ages can do it. Whether you are young or old, the pool is ready for you. Not only can swimming strengthen your heart and lungs, it also strengthens your core muscles, which includes your hips. Swimming is very good for those who are recovering from a hip flexor injury. Since your body is able to float in the water, swimming is an exercise that is much easier on your hips than running or biking. You can even walk in the water to warm-up. If you are not into strength training exercises, you can substitute it with swimming but be sure to warm up and stretch before you go in.

Stretches for Hip Rehabilitation

After you warm up, it is important to properly stretch your muscles before engaging in any type of exercise. Stretching before you exercise is important because it can help improve your range of motion and it can also help prevent future injuries. Stretching after you exercise can help decrease muscle soreness and can keep them flexible.

The first stretch you can do is the **standing iliotibial band stretch.** To start, you will need to stand near a wall. Then, take the foot that is closest to the wall and cross it over your other foot. Next, move your hip toward the wall to stretch it. Stay like that for 30 seconds. You can do this 4 times for each leg in two sets.

Try to do this stretch once a day. To see a visual of this stretch, please check out the YouTube video Iliotibial Band Stretch by FitnessBlender.

The second stretch you can do is the **seated rotation stretch**. To do this, sit on the floor and stretch your legs out in front of you. Cross one of your legs over the other one and slowly twist your upper body toward the leg that is bent. You can put your hand behind you to support yourself. Put your other hand on your bent leg and gently stretch yourself a little further. To fully stretch your hip, look over your shoulder and allow yourself to stretch for half a minute. Slowly bring yourself back and return to your original position. You can do this 4 times in 2 sets. Try to do this stretch once a day.

The third stretch you can do is the **knee to chest stretch.** To do this, lay on the ground and stretch your legs out. Bend one leg and hold your shin with your hands. Gently pull your leg toward your chest but do not force it. Hold it for 30 seconds and then return to your original position. Do the same for the other leg and then do it once with both legs at a time. You can do this 2 times in 4 sets. Try to do this stretch once a day. For a visual of this stretch, please check out Thespinesolution's YouTube video knee to chest stretch.

The fourth stretch you can do is the **supine hamstring stretch.** To start, lie on the ground and bend both of your knees. Lift one leg up to a 90 degree angle. Grasp the back of your upper thighs with your hand. Slowly pull your leg forward until you can feel it stretch. Allow yourself to stretch for 30 seconds and then release. Do the same process for your other leg and complete 2 full sets of 4 repetitions. Try to do this stretch once a day. To see this stretch in action, please check out this YouTube video, Leg Exercise – Supine Hamstring Stretch, by Pain Therapy.

Strength Training Exercises For Hip Rehabilitation

Once you have finished stretching, you can move on to strength exercises. Strength training after a hip injury can help relieve pain and strengthen your hip joints against new injuries.

The first strength rehabilitation exercise you can begin with is a **hip abduction.** Lie on your side, keeping your injured side up and your strong side on the bottom. Relax your top leg and gently raise it until it is situated at 45 degrees. Stay like that for 5 seconds and then release. Give yourself 2 seconds and repeat. Do 8 repetitions on each side at least 3 days a week. You can optionally add weight for increased resistance. To see this exercise in action, please check out this YouTube video by Mid-Columbia Medical Center, PT Exercise –Hip Abduction.

The second strength rehabilitation exercise you can begin with is a **hip adduction.** Lie on the ground, injured leg down. Cross the top leg over your bottom leg. Next, raise your bottom leg between 6 and 8 inches off the floor.

Keep your leg up for 5 seconds and then bring it down and rest. Repeat this exercise 8 times on both sides for at least 3 days a week. You can optionally add a weight for increased resistance. To see this exercise in action, please check out this YouTube video, Hip Adduction Exercise by Rocky Mountain Pediatric Orthopedic.

The third strength rehabilitation exercise you can begin with is a **hip extension**. Put a pillow beneath your hips and lay down on your stomach. Bend one of your knees at a 90 degree angle and allow your leg to lift up, pointing toward the ceiling. While counting to five, slowly lower your leg back down. Repeat this exercise 8 times per leg for 3 days a week.

The fourth strength rehabilitation exercise you can begin with is an **internal hip rotation.** Lie comfortably on your side with a pillow in between your upper legs. Cross your top leg over your body and let your foot hang over the side of a table or bed. Next, lift your foot as high as possible and begin to rotate your hips while counting to five, and then slowly return to your original position. You can do this 8 times for each side and should be done 3 days a week.

Chapter 6: Staying Motivated

If you've incurred a hip injury it is likely that you will need to go through some physical therapy and rehabilitation to allow your injury to heal. While everybody enjoys having some downtime, spending time resting and rehabbing your body can become pretty depressing, especially if you're used to being up, about, and active. Many people often fall into depression and become angry since they are unable to go about their normal routine. However, by staying motivated and upbeat during your rehab process, you can help your hips heal even quicker. This chapter will provide you with some ideas and tips on how to do so.

Visualizing Positive Thoughts

One of the easiest and physically effortless ways to get through rehabbing your hips is to stay positive. The more negative thoughts you have the more unhappy your life can be. One thing you can do to pass time and heal your injury is to think about what you want to do with yourself when you're ready to get back on your feet. Spend your downtime reflecting on what goals you'd like to set for yourself and think about ways you can achieve them. Visualize yourself in the position that you'd like to be in and it can help keep you motivated to get there. You can even take your downtime as a challenge—it can help you strengthen your mind so that you will be a stronger person for the future. If you need to sharpen your skills on staying motivated and determined to reach your goals, please check out my book Influence, Willpower, and Discipline. One trick to visualization is to make the pictures in your mind appear as if you're watching yourself from above or on a TV screen. Also, too much visualization of a positive outcome can sometimes actually convince your brain that you have already achieved your goal and therefore become a little demotivating. So a good strategy is to visualize yourself going through the rehab process itself and then visualizing the positive results at the end.

Learn Something New

If you have to be confined to your house for a little bit, view it as an opportunity to learn something new. You can read a book, try your hand at a new hobby, or even watch an interesting documentary on TV. You can learn to draw, paint, play an instrument, or a variety of different things. The choices are endless. Find something that interests you and immerse yourself in it to keep your spirits high. Learning something new will keep you busy and help the time that it will take you to recover fly by. For more ideas on using your spare time productively, be sure to check out my book: Ultimate Productivity.

Look Forward to Physical Therapy

If you're recovering from a hip injury, it is likely that you will need to spend some time in a physical therapist's office. Use this opportunity to make a new friend as you sit in the waiting room. You may even end up finding somebody who you can connect with and workout with afterwards. I always like to say that there is something good in everything, even if it's a little discouraging. You may even ask your physical therapist to play your favorite music during your exercises. Listening to your favorite music can help you stay upbeat and positive throughout each session.

Get Help From Family and Friends

Not being able to go about your daily life may have a hindering effect on your social life. If you can't go see your family and friends, you can consider asking them to come see you. Spending time with your loved ones is a great way to make time fly. You can laugh together, joke with each other, and just keep each other company. You will also feel great knowing that you have a strong support system behind you.

Hypnosis

Some people may turn to hypnosis to get through their rehabilitation process. At Hypnosis Downloads, you can have access to some of the best hypnosis resources. You can find resources to help you fight depression, enjoy life, overcome physical pain, and how to stay motivated and inspired. Listening to one or two hypnosis downloads a day would definitely be an intelligent way to maximize your rehab process.

Don't Rush

Most importantly, do not rush your rehabilitation process. If you rush, you may end up damaging your injury further and you will be out of commission for even longer than you first expected. Take it slow, day by day, and you will do just fine. Make sure that you are able to communicate well with your doctors or therapists if you are still in pain or if you feel uncomfortable doing any of the exercises. Do not let your injury take control over you. Make your rehab the most important thing that you do each day, and just be sure to do everything correctly. If you commit yourself totally to healing your injury you will be better before you know it!

Conclusion

I hope this book was able to help you to learn about the importance of keeping your hips strong and in shape as well as how to protect them during and after an injury or deteriorating condition.

The next step is to start working some of the stretches and exercises that this book has covered into your daily routine. The sooner you start taking care of your hips, the less chance that you will have problems with them in the future. If you end up injuring them or know somebody who has injured them, you now know exactly what needs to be done. Finally, keep the chapter on staying motivated in mind, even if you do not have to go through a rehabilitation process. Staying motivated and positive is the key to getting through life happy and healthy!

Finally, if you discovered at least one thing that has helped you or that you think would be beneficial to someone else, be sure to take a few seconds to easily post a quick positive review. As an author, your positive feedback is desperately needed. Your highly valuable five star reviews are like a river of golden joy flowing through a sunny forest of mighty trees and beautiful flowers! *To do your good deed in making the world a better place by helping others with your valuable insight, just leave a nice review.*

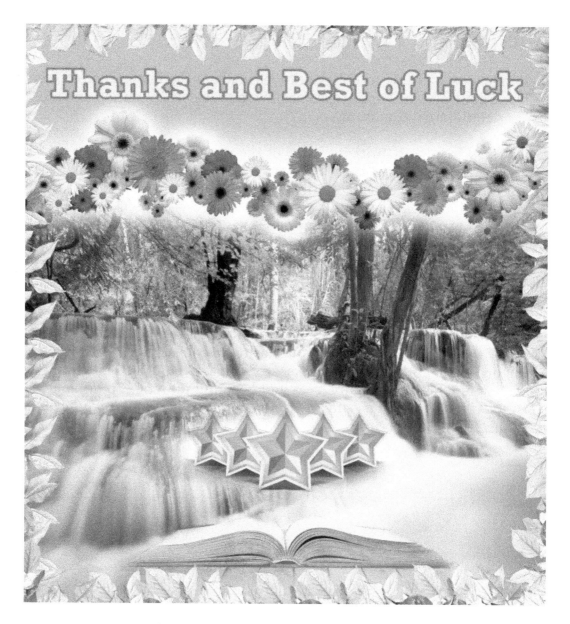

My Other Books and Audio Books
www.AcesEbooks.com

Health Books

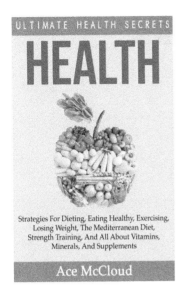

ULTIMATE HEALTH SECRETS

HEALTH

Strategies For Dieting, Eating Healthy, Exercising,
Losing Weight, The Mediterranean Diet,
Strength Training, And All About Vitamins,
Minerals, And Supplements

Ace McCloud

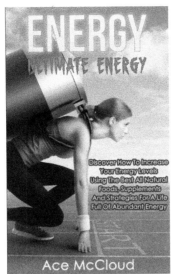

ENERGY
ULTIMATE ENERGY

Discover How To Increase
Your Energy Levels
Using The Best All Natural
Foods, Supplements
And Strategies For A Life
Full Of Abundant Energy

Ace McCloud

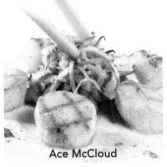

RECIPE BOOK

The Best Food Recipes
That Are Delicious, Healthy,
Great For Energy And Easy To Make

Ace McCloud

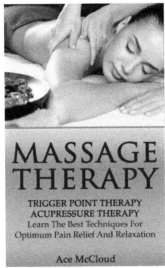

MASSAGE
THERAPY

TRIGGER POINT THERAPY
ACUPRESSURE THERAPY
Learn The Best Techniques For
Optimum Pain Relief And Relaxation

Ace McCloud

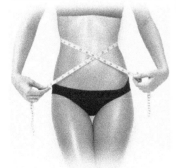

LOSE WEIGHT

THE TOP 100 BEST WAYS
TO LOSE WEIGHT QUICKLY AND HEALTHILY

Ace McCloud

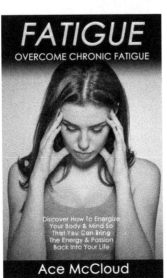

FATIGUE
OVERCOME CHRONIC FATIGUE

Discover How To Energize
Your Body & Mind So
That You Can Bring
The Energy & Passion
Back Into Your Life

Ace McCloud

Peak Performance Books

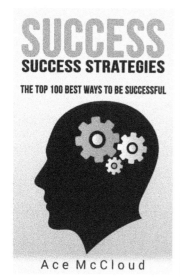

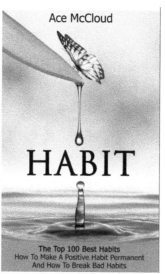

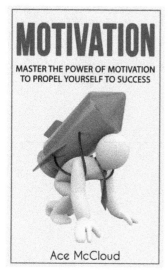

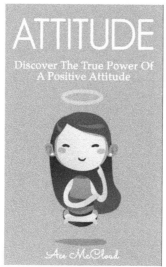

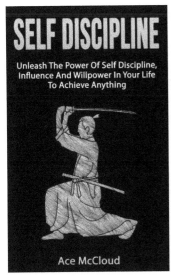
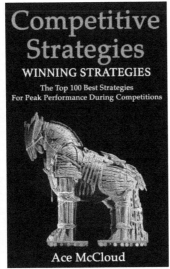

Be sure to check out my audio books as well!

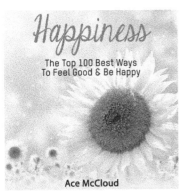
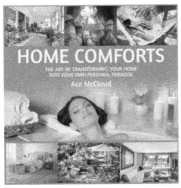
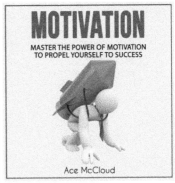

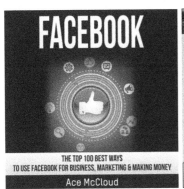
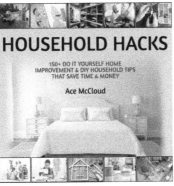
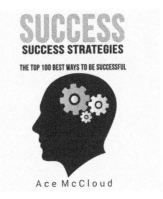

Check out my website at: **www.AcesEbooks.com** for a complete list of all of my books and high quality audio books. I enjoy bringing you the best knowledge in the world and wish you the best in using this information to make your journey through life better and more enjoyable! **Best of luck to you!**

CPSIA information can be obtained
at www.ICGtesting.com
Printed in the USA
BVHW010622080119
537203BV00017BA/1882/P